# THE MYSTERY OF LIFE

## BLOOD ON MY HANDS ....BLOOD IN THE LAND

Revealing the spiritual Implications of Abortion/Blood and Fertility
Options for Couples Desiring Children

Including thorny questions like "can Christians undergo
surrogacy?","What does God say about IVF?"

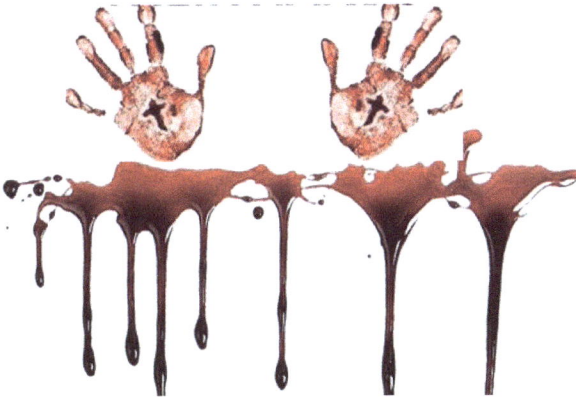

By

**Nelly Nelly**

Published by Hemingway Publishers

Cover design by Hemingway Publishers

ISBN: Printed in the United States

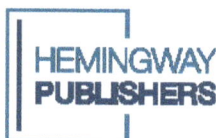

HEMINGWAY
PUBLISHERS

2

# FOREWORD

With the unabated number of abortions and other fertility issues around the
ld, I am compelled to share invaluable insights into the significance of blood
. is laid in my heart after long years of study, personal experiences, and divine
ction in this regard.

Although different religions may have their perspectives on these issues,
ertheless, the author draws deep insights and truths from the Christian
spective – specifically the Bible.

I encourage every single, married, or prospective parent to read the hidden
sures of this book. It took lots of courage for me to pen this down and to release
) the public because it draws from my personal experiences and with others as
l, which was difficult for me to share but which I know would be a lifesaver to
neone out there.

The actual names of those who shared their lived experiences are
livulged due to Confidentiality.

Giving back to humanity in diverse forms has always been my desire. Come
)ard as we plunge into revelations of a deep trend the world has called modern
: in which the Lord intends to intervene.

# TABLE OF CONTENTS

# INTRODUCTION

Dora[1] was a beautiful, boisterous girl who dropped out of High School ause she was the breadwinner of her home with a mother and siblings to care She took on that role at a tender age, so it was really worrisome to hear her n calling her incessantly to transfer some money home to meet some basic ds. One would wonder what job her mum thinks she does to get money. On the er hand, she was estranged from family and friends, cohabiting with her friend, whose sisters had chased her out because she was pregnant with him for fourth time.

She was now in a transit home and had vowed that this time she would not e in to removing the baby, but every night, she would cry her eyes out as she ened to her boyfriend chide and taunt her never to keep the child. A little more ) to counsel the young man revealed he could not put up with her because he felt mother was a troublesome woman, as acclaimed. Concerning the many rtions she had undergone for him, he claimed he could not vouch for her hfulness; besides, they had broken up, and he was planning on marrying another who, to him, was more decent. Nothing would ever make him feel tied down another girl. Somehow, she eventually had a miscarriage that left everyone king if she took a pill or not due to the pressure.

Thelma, another young girl, had just finished her University Education and s undergoing her Master's Degree when she stumbled upon a young man who s working at a good job. He professed his love was always at her beck and call, Alas! She got pregnant; the young man stopped picking up her calls and

---

[1] All names are not the real names of the clients. Ethically, all the personal details of clients are kept confidential. However, all events are true life experiences of those who have given their consent to share their stories in documents/books.

suddenly became too busy to visit her again. She ran to the transit home. W[hat] would she do? She is a Christian worker in the church, and she attends Bible Sch[ool]. She is preparing to be ordained as a pastor soon in the campus church. She [was] counseled to embrace life for her Unborn and also encouraged with her religi[ous] compass (the Bible) for direction, showing different scriptures that supported [a] course of life.

'What would be the point of your ordination if you grieve the Holy Spi[rit]? Two wrongs don't make a right," – the counselor had asked her. For a while, [she] agreed to keep the baby. She was enrolled in pre-natal classes in one of the g[ood] hospitals in town. However, one fateful Sunday night, she called that she w[as] bleeding. A little probe would reveal that her religious mentor counseled her agai[nst] keeping the baby. The mentor asked her – 'You will soon be ordained, rememb[er]. What would the church say?' She gave in to the pressure.

These two extreme stories mirror the challenges of many young girls [out] there who are unable to speak up against Gender-based Violence and socie[tal] pressures to accept abortion.

**How Pregnancy Occurs**

When there is an onset of menstruation, it is presumed that a girl can [get] pregnant. In simple terms, a girl who has started ovulating can get pregnant wh[en] she is sexually intimate with a fertile man. During this process, millions of spe[rm] cells are released by the male into the cervix of the female. These sperm cells sw[im] rapidly through the fallopian tube, searching for the egg/ovum that is usua[lly] released monthly from a woman's ovaries. When found, the sperm cells dig into [the] ovum. Still, only one sperm reaches the pronuclei of the ovum and fuses toget[her] with it, fertilizes the ovum, and a fetus is formed through a process that eventua[lly] travels down to the uterus to implant and grows into a baby.

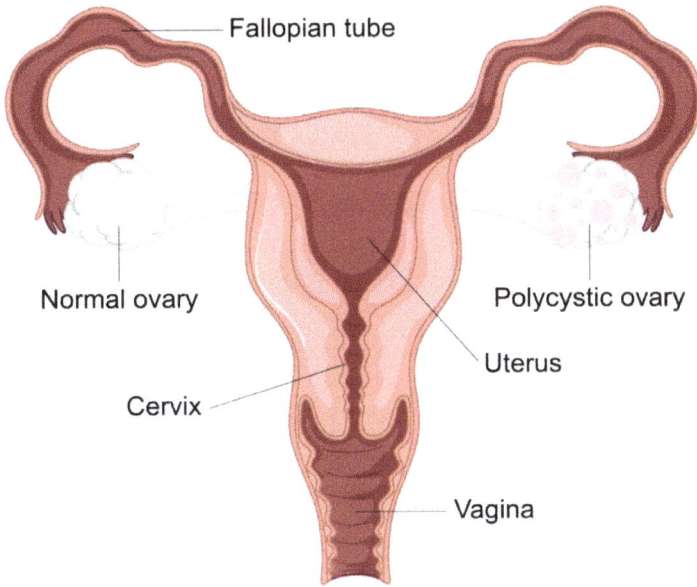

Fallopian tube

Normal ovary

Polycystic ovary

Cervix

Uterus

Vagina

In many countries, when an unplanned pregnancy occurs, a lady might de to terminate the pregnancy, which is called an abortion – spilling the blood n innocent, vulnerable baby. Sparing the life of the child is recommended.

# 1. Ways People Spill Blood

Blood is spilled when persons kill or cut short the life of another human being, especially when it is done intentionally.

Someone can have blood on their hands when they refuse to share information that God has specifically told them to – *"If I say to the wicked, 'shall surely die,' and you give him no warning, nor speak to warn the wicked from his wicked way, in order to save his life, that wicked person shall die for iniquity, but his blood I will require at your hand."(Ezekiel 3:18, ESV).*

**What is Abortion?**

Biologically, there are four *main* stages of an unborn human: *zygote* (from conception to 4-5 days); *blastocyst* (from 5 days to implantation in the uterine wall about nine days); *embryo* (from implantation to the first sign of brain waves—about eight weeks); *fetus* (from about eight weeks to birth).   Often, in non-medical settings, the term 'fetus' is used to cover all stages.

Abortion is the expulsion of the fetus from the womb before it has reached a stage where it can survive outside the mother. It can occur spontaneously, in which case it is called a *miscarriage*. It can also be brought on purposefully for medical or social reasons, in which case it is called an *induced abortion*. For this book, would refer to induced abortion plainly as abortion.

Abortion can be performed through various means, which include taking certain drugs orally or inserting them into the vagina, taking nicotine, hard drugs, herbal concoctions, dilatation and curettage (D&C), manual vacuum aspiration (MVA), etc.

All but a few countries allow abortion for one or more of the following ...sons: To protect the life of the woman, to protect her physical or mental health, ...ases of rape or sexual abuse, Serious fetal anomaly, Socioeconomic reasons, ...at the woman's request. These reasons could be subject to objective reasoning, ...hown in the study below.

# 2. Abortion Prevalence

According to the Guttmacher Institute (2022), 121 million uninten
pregnancies worldwide were recorded annually between 2015 and 2019, with u
73 million ending in abortion (61%). Abortion rates were prevalent across l
income, middle, and high-income Countries, with middle-income countries top
the chart at 66%. Although more unintended pregnancies occurred in Count
where there were abortion restrictions, these restrictions influenced the uptake
abortions as abortions were significantly lower (49%) compared to Countries wh
it was legal (70%).

# 3. Medical mitigations of Abortion

Abstinence from sexual intercourse and the use of effective contraceptives the two most effective means of personal prevention of unwanted pregnancy. ny pregnant girls who, amidst pressures, decide to keep their babies lack the uisite social support system in many societies to make them pull through. The st hit are those in low and middle-income countries with little or no safety nets :ater to their needs. Within this period, they are estranged from family and nds, with little or no financial support, and in dire need of entrepreneurial skills elp them sustain themselves and the babies upon delivery. It is on this premise : adoption and maternity transit homes gained their relevance as they care for neless pregnant young women to curb the menace of illegal human and child ficking and infant and maternal mortality due to unsafe abortions.

**Why is Abortion – Murder?**

**Blood!!! What exactly is the big deal about Blood?**

Blood represents life (Leviticus 17:11 For the life of a creature is in the od, and I have given it to you to make atonement for yourselves on the altar; it he blood that makes atonement for one's life) and can be used as a ransom. As ney is the legal tender here on earth to obtain goods and services, so is blood in spiritual realm to obtain ransom. When Adam and Eve sinned, they covered mselves with leaves. Still, God knew it was not sufficient to cover their iritual) nakedness, so for the first time, an animal was killed, and the blood ned for man's sins temporarily before God used the skin of the animal to cover ir nakedness fully. Eventually, the lamb would be the most potent substitute *evelation 13:8And all that dwell upon the earth shall worship him, whose names : not written in* **the Book of Life** *of the Lamb, slain from the foundation of the rld.)*

Medically, a living organism means – an organism that is alive. Liv[...] organisms are composed of cells. They divide and begin to multiply as a sign[...] growth. Organisms grow after their kind, so a human organism means tha[...] conception, a human being different from the father and mother is already grow[...] as evidenced by the embryo going through cellular division and expansion.

Biblically, God regards the soul of a human being, which exists even bef[...] the embryo (which is the body) is formed *(Jeremiah 1:5a: "Before I formed yo[...] the womb, I knew you, before you were born, I set you apart;)* how much more w[...] that soul has been physically conceived in an embryo form, hence God sees one-minute or one-day-old embryo as a living Human being as seen in

*Psalm 139: 13-16: For you created my inmost being; you knit me toget[...] in my mother's womb. I praise you because I am fearfully and wonderfully ma[...] your works are wonderful; I know that full well. My frame was not hidden from y[...] when I was made in the secret place when I was woven together in the depths of[...] earth. Your eyes **saw my unformed body**; all the days ordained for me were writ[...] in your book before one of them came to be.*

*Psalm 51:5:Surely I was sinful at birth, sinful from the time my mot[...] conceived me.*

"Exodus 21:22 If people are fighting and hit a pregnant woman and s[...] gives birth prematurely[e] but there is no serious injury, the offender must be fin[...] whatever the woman's husband demands and the court allows. ²³ But if there[...] serious injury, you are to take life for life, ²⁴ eye for eye, tooth for tooth, hand [...] hand, foot for foot, ²⁵ burn for burn, wound for wound, bruise for bruise.

(The serious injury here means that either the unborn baby or the wom[...] dies; if this is so, the Mosaic law had commanded death in return).

For a lady who gets pregnant and is under intense pressure to terminate the nancy, the Lord is saying in **Deuteronomy 30:19**: *This day I call the heavens the earth as witnesses against you that I have set before you life and death, sings and curses. Now, choose life so that you and your children (seed, endants) may live.*

Remember that in the New Testament order, mostly ceremonial laws were awed by Jesus Christ's death, but moral laws such as murder are still upheld, cially spiritually.

### Could this be a Doomsday Message?

God is a loving Father and does not want us to serve him in fear, for There o fear in love. But perfect love drives out fear because fear has to do with ishment. The one who fears is not made perfect in love. (1 John 4:18). There is vine mystery of love – the Father'slove for a generation of young people who be confused, alone, developing a sense of low self-worth, and who lack ntorship and sound moral guidance.

Living in a society full of stigma for the sinful and a desire to stone the lteress woman, this area of work has remained fallow over the years with no to seek the straying and those who have been raped or involved in sexual norality. One thing stands sure: "Eze.33:11: Tell them that as surely as I, the ereign LORD, am the living God, I do not enjoy seeing sinners die. I would rather them stop sinning and live".For those who fall through the cracks and get gnant, we encourage life for both the unborn and the mother. Due to a shortage social safety nets for these groups of girls, many have taken to abortion, child ficking, poor maternal/neonatal health, illegal adoption, and selling of their ies, forgetting that at some point in life, a mother's love cries out for her child.

Unfortunately, in a world full of stigma for the unmarried pregnant there are enough reasons to want to consider abortion, such as rape, having a c out of wedlock, irresponsibility of the partner, shame, strict/religious pare poverty/inability to care for the child, teenage pregnancy, the need to pursue o studies/further education, cultural reasons and peer pressure. Still, after read through the experiences of others, one may need to reconsider if these reasons worth the life of that baby. God's condemnation of abortion does not mean doesn't love the mother. We can fully enjoy all that God wills for us if we obey injunctions. God had earlier commanded, "You must show no pity for the gu Your rule should be life for life, eye for eye, tooth for tooth, hand for hand, foot foot. (Deut.19:21) and later, "The Wages of Sin is Death, but the gift of Go eternal life in Christ Jesus our Lord"(Rom.6:23).

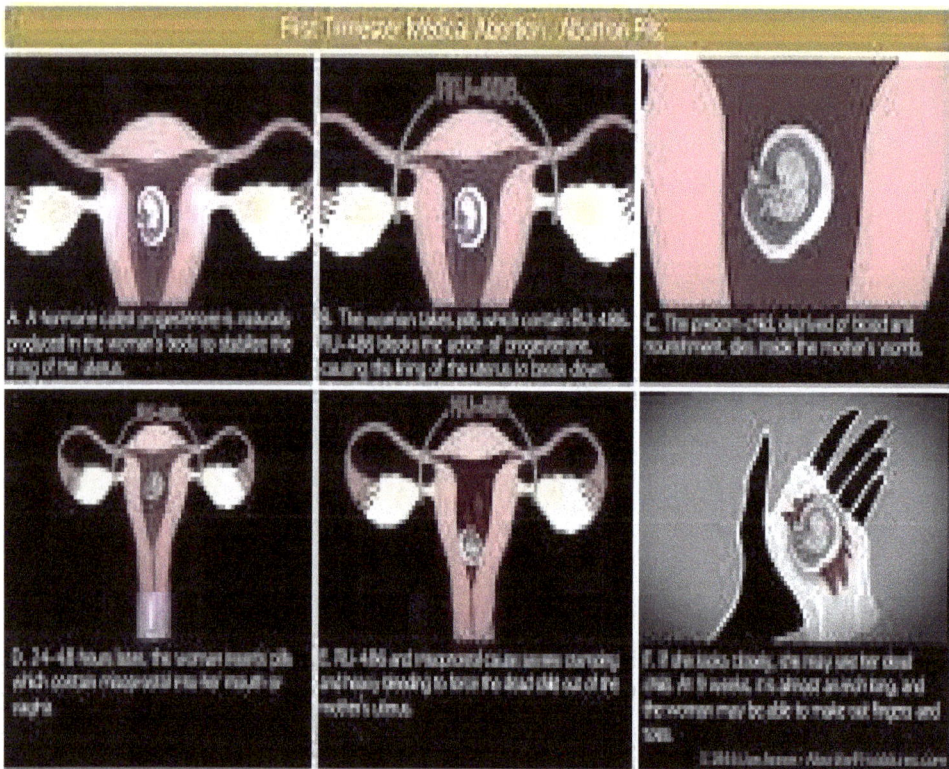

In battle, men are allowed to defend themselves, and the death of a man is sidered murder if he has no opportunity to defend himself. Every fetus is first ocent of the mistakes of their parents. Secondly, they are so fragile that they end on their mother for survival, protection, and growth. How grievous it is en the same person that has been designed to protect suddenly becomes the tor, the very one to rip off the baby from the womb in death.

# Types of Abortion

Medical Abortion is done by taking oral pills that are capable of interfe**r**
with the hormone –progesterone, which is responsible for making the pregna**n**
grow. It also stops the flow of nutrients and eventually induces an abortion. W**h**
an abortion pill is taken, it cuts off the flow of nutrients from the

mother to the baby, and after some time, the baby dies. After that, ano**t**
pill that induces abortion is taken to expel the dead baby. Sometimes, an or**a**
induced abortion may not completely expel all the remains from the uterus, ar**d**
D&C or MVA may still be required to clear all contents.

## Surgical Abortion

1. **Dilation and curettage (D&C)** refers to the dilation (widening/opening**)**
   the cervix and surgical removal of part of the lining of the uterus or conte**nts**
   of the uterus by scraping and scooping (curettage). It is usually done in
   first trimester. It is also used as a therapeutic gynecological procedure.
2. Dilatation and Evacuation: This refers to the dilation of the cervix **and**
   removal of the baby using narrow forceps passed through the cervix. I**t is**
   usually done between 15 and 24 weeks of pregnancy.
3. Vacuum Aspiration: The fetus is removed by gentle suction, which can **be**
   done manually or electronically. It is usually done for pregnancies in **the**
   first trimester.

# HOW IS AN ABORTION PICTORIALLY DONE?

## Suction and Curettage Abortion of a 9 Week Old Fetus

A. A speculum is placed in the vagina, a tenaculum is clamped to the lip of the cervix and a cannula is inserted into the uterus.

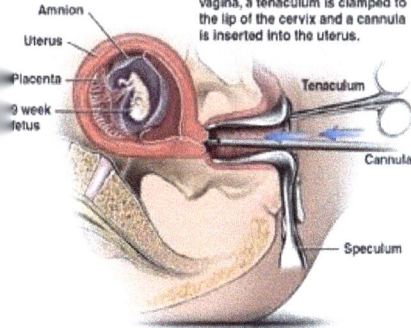

Amnion
Uterus
Placenta
9 week fetus
Tenaculum
Cannula
Speculum

Cut-away view of mother's pelvis

B. The amniotic fluid, placenta and fetus are suctioned through the cannula into a collection jar. The fetus and placenta are torn apart in the process.

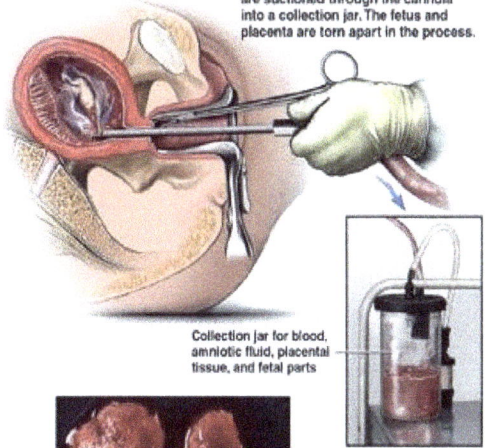

Collection jar for blood, amniotic fluid, placental tissue, and fetal parts

C. The uterine cavity is scraped with a curette to determine whether any significant amount of tissue remains.

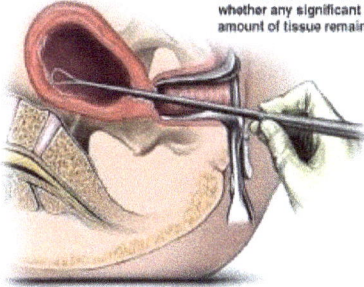

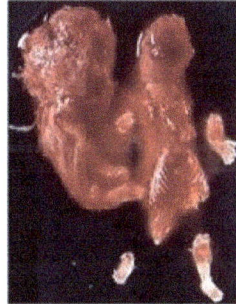

D. The contents of the collection jar are examined to assure that all fetal parts and an adequate amount of tissue commensurate with estimated gestational age are present.

# Dilation and Evacuation Abortion (D&E) of a 23 Week Old Fetus

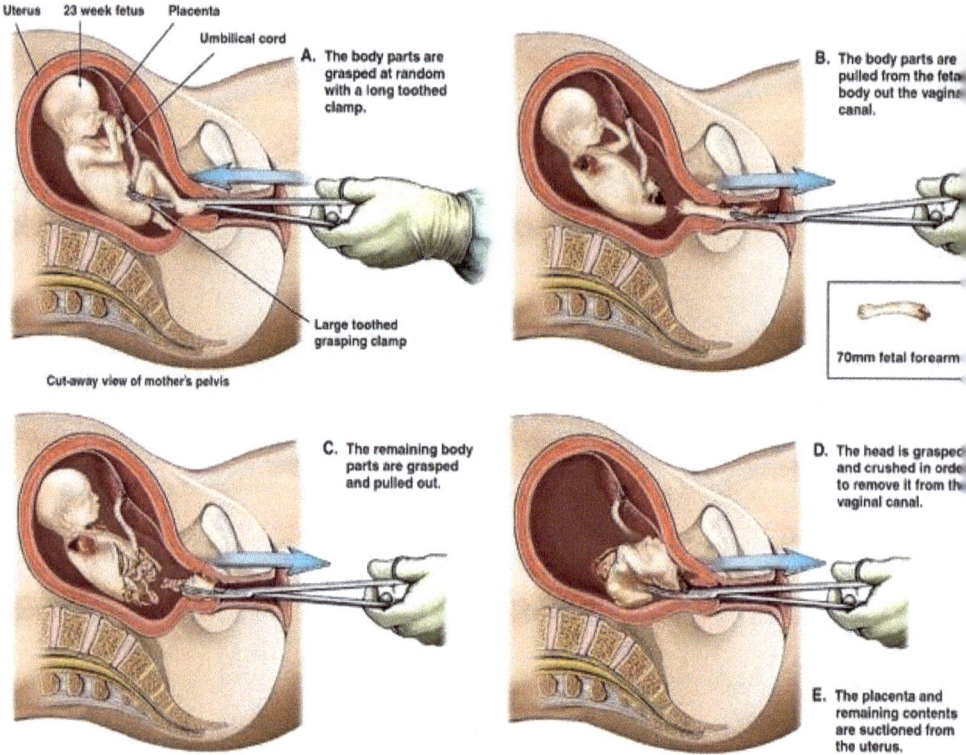

Uterus    23 week fetus    Placenta

Umbilical cord

A. The body parts are grasped at random with a long toothed clamp.

B. The body parts are pulled from the fetal body out the vaginal canal.

Large toothed grasping clamp

Cut-away view of mother's pelvis

70mm fetal forearm

C. The remaining body parts are grasped and pulled out.

D. The head is grasped and crushed in order to remove it from the vaginal canal.

E. The placenta and remaining contents are suctioned from the uterus.

Most clinicians recommend an abortion in the first twelve (12) weeks pregnancy because they believe the fetus is not fully formed, but this does not make it less of a murder case. Worse still are couples or girls who still insist terminating a pregnancy later than 12 weeks and some well into the third trimester. Observe below the physiology of a fetus below 12 weeks.

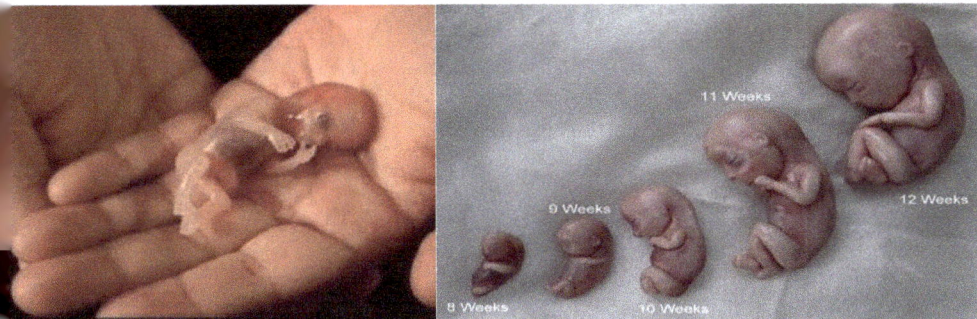

In a cross-section of fetal beings below 12 weeks, there is the presence
' a head, limbs, and, most importantly, a heartbeat. The earliest a fetal
:artbeat can be detected is at 6weeks of pregnancy. Literally speaking, that is
ıly two weeks after a girl misses her period/menstrual flow

## How are terminated fetuses disposed of?

Many times, especially in countries where abortion is illegal, many ladies
ıng for elective abortion never really see the remains of their babies nor choose
ıt happens to them after that. In the United Kingdom, they have banned the
:eration and sluicing (the fetuses are melted with acidic substances or using a
:eration machine to beat the fetus to pulp, separating the pulp from fluid and
ı flushing through a passageway for easier disposal) of fetal remains and instead
•pted the selective disposal guidelines where the remains are placed in a jar and
ɔosed in a separate waste bin different from bins used in collecting other medical
ite to honor the sanctity of the terminated life. In many countries, there are no
ct guidelines concerning the disposal of elective terminated fetuses, meaning
t hospitals may just decide to discard terminated fetuses in the general bin, melt
m with acid, flush them down the toilet, or throw them into a drainage without

being penalized. This exacerbates the cruelty of a young life, being terminated not given a proper burial.

## Complications of Abortion

Abortion, even when carried out in a safe environment, can lead to a var of complications, which could be minor or major.

## Minor Complications

1. Pain
2. Mild bleeding
3. Infection
4. Post anesthesia complications

## Major Complications

1. Heavy bleeding, which could be life-threatening
2. Injury to the uterus
3. Injury to the bladder or intestines
4. Injury to the cervix, which can cause difficulty in subsequent deliveries
5. Failed abortion
6. Septic abortion (a generalized infection that occurs as a result of process)
7. Infertility is a result of scar formation in the uterus, which impedes or blo the uterine cavity.

## 6. Sacredness of Blood – Historical accounts.

"Anyone who strikes a person with a fatal blow is to be put to death.[13] ~vever, if it is not done intentionally, but God lets it happen, they are to flee to a ~e I will designate.[14] But if anyone schemes and kills someone deliberately, that ~son is to be taken from my altar and put to death. (Exo.21:12-14)

- Adam and Eve

In the beginning, God made the heavens and the earth; he made all animals, ~ the first man and woman were Adam and Eve. Animals and Man cohabited ~cefully without hurting each other. Everyone ate from the Garden of Eden. ~re were enough fruit-bearing Trees to feed both Man and Animals. However, ~d instructed Adam in Genesis 2:16 – *"You may eat the fruit of any tree in the ~den* (Enough Provision)*, except the tree that gives knowledge of what is good ~l what is bad* (First warning)*. You must not eat the fruit of the tree* (Second ~rning)*; if you do, you will die* (Spiritual death) *the same day (*and eventually ~sical death)."* How often does God encourage us to be satisfied in His abundant ~vision of peace found in righteous living and warn us through our parents, ~ardians, loved ones, and Spiritual leaders to stay away from sin, especially ~ual immorality – what is our response to these warnings?

Adam and Eve did not just follow their instincts. They gave deep thought ~their actions after the devil tempted them – *"The Woman saw how beautiful the ~e was and how good its fruit would be to eat, and she **thought** how wonderful it ~uld be to become wise, so she took some of the fruit and ate it, ... and he (Adam) ~o ate (Gen.3:6).* How many times have you considered how curvy, beautiful and ~nderful that girl is, how intensely you spend hours thinking how it would be to ~ld her in your arms and intimately have sex with her. How many times have you ~d down on your bed thinking how nice that boy/man is, how his big strong arms

can carry you, tenderly kiss you, and how you could reciprocate all his kindnes
you – who knows, you both may end up in marriage. Gradually, we spend m
time with them, hold hands, and start smooching – it's not so bad, we think,
somehow, we end up in sexual impurity.

Adam and Eve eventually ate the fruit, but what came after was far fr
their thoughts. They realized how naked they were (Gen.3: 7), *so they sewed*
*leaves together and covered themselves.* They were so afraid of God's presen
couldn't stand his voice, Him passing by, how much more beholding His fac
Impossible. How badly our consciences beat us up after that first kiss, that f
masturbation, and that first sex. It was far away from our initial thoughts. It soun
so good when we watched it on television or on the Internet, but it was not
pleasant as we thought. We lose our peace, our relationship with God dies, and
are sometimes faced with a Sexually Transmitted Infection/HIV, Pregnancy, d
out from school, and the pains of childbirth are all too much pain that we did
think about before the act. Our thoughts focused too much on the pleasures of
but not the consequences of our actions. For the first couple, the woman would ha
to go through intense pain at childbirth, the man would till the hard ground to fe
and they would constantly be in enmity with the serpent. Thereafter, they wo
never live in peace with other wild animals anymore.

And for the first time, blood had to be spilled – an animal was killed, a
God removed the skin of the animal to cover up Man's nakedness (*Gen.3:21 – A*
*the Lord God made clothes out of animal skins for Adam and his Wife, and*
*clothed them*). God is still telling us today that someone must need to die (spiritua
and physically) anytime we sin (*For the Wages of Sin is Death – Romans 6:23*
Adam and Eve were lucky to have an animal die physically for them to cover (
take away) their sin – what about you? Who would you present to die for your S

ny girls always think that taking that contraceptive pill or killing that unborn
d would further cover their sexual sins, but does it take the Sin AWAY?

*"Whoever sheds man's blood, By man his blood shall be shed, For in the
ge of God He made man. Genesis 9:6*

## Cain and Abel

In Genesis 4, somehow, God yearned for a (blood) sacrifice. Could it be that
am and Eve's Sin continued to speak that even when an animal was killed to
er their nakedness, God still yearned for a sacrifice because Hebrews 10:4 says
*blood of bulls and goats can't take away sins.* Even though it was required yearly
atone for the sins of men in the Levitical times (Heb.9:7). In response, Abel (a
ephard) offered the first lamb born to one of his sheep and sacrificed the best part
God ...*The Lord was pleased with **ABEL and his offering, but he rejected CAIN
farmer) and his offering (harvested from his plants/farm) because** it lacked*
**od**. It is important to note that God was first pleased with the person of Abel
ore accepting his sacrifice. And God had rejected the person of Cain even before
offered his vain sacrifice. How many times do we try to get busy in the name of
ORK to bring our tithes and offerings to God when we are first living sinful lives,
do these works lack blood? They add no value to the lives or salvation of men.
display our evil intents and cunning attitudes to make a profit. Our characters
stained with pride, spite, and sensual behavior to lead men to sin. We seek to
ss our examinations by hook or crook, never giving a minute to share God's love
a dying world through our words and characters. God is pleased with Shepherds,
se who find an opportunity to minister God's word through their work and
ions so men can be saved. Men and women who will not frivolously play with
quity, masturbation, lesbianism, smooching, kissing, indecent dressing, and
tful lucre but apply 1 Cor.7:9: "*But if they cannot control themselves, they should*

*marry, for it is better to marry than to burn with passion."* Matt 5:28: *"But I tell that anyone who looks at a woman lustfully has already committed adultery with her in his heart."* Many ladies and men find it interesting, as sport or fun, to gain sexual attention of the opposite sex. They would dress to kill, take long walks the street even at night, spend long hours with the opposite sex in ungodly hours watch pornographic materials, read heavily sensual novels, visit the opposite alone in lonely places, or even engage in same-sex sexual exploration. All su behaviors can make us rejected in God's sight. You may not have actually physical sex, but by merely condoning these behaviors and defiling your heart you can be rejected. It was difficult for Prophet Samuel to understand, for when was to anoint a King in Israel as he went searching in the house of Jesse, he co vouch that he could see Kingly qualities in the person of Eliab – Jesse's first So Outwardly, he could pass for a King but Alas!!

*"But the Lord said to Samuel, 'Do not consider his appearance or his heig for I have rejected him. The Lord does not look at the things people look at. Peo look at the outward appearance, but the Lord looks at the heart". (1 Sam.16:7).*

Understanding that it is important to guard our hearts diligently, for out it flows the issues of life (Prv.4:23). Instead of repenting, some still behave l: Cain when corrected –

*"Why are you angry? Why that scowl on your face? If you had done right thing, you would be smiling, but because you have done evil, sin is crouch at your door. It wants to rule you, but you must overcome it." (Gen.4:6-7)*

If you do not repent from acts that defile your heart, you may eventua engage in sexual immorality.

Cain refused to repent. He lured Abel to the fields and killed him - the fi human murder occurred – The blood of Abel began speaking against his broth

Cain was punished in Gen.4: 10-16 with a curse, unprofitability, ‹elessness/wanderer, and finally spiritual death (Gen.4:16 – *Cain went away ‹ the Lord's presence.*).

"Then the Lord said, 'Why have you done this terrible thing? Your brother's ‹d is crying out to me from the ground, like a voice calling for revenge.'"

**BLOOD SPEAKS;** it can either speak vengeance as in the case of Abel or ‹k mercy as in the case of our Lord Jesus Christ

"*You have come to Jesus, the one who mediates the new covenant between ‹ and people, and to the sprinkled blood, which speaks of forgiveness instead of ‹ng out for vengeance like the blood of Abel (*Heb.12:24 – NLT)

For many who might have crossed the line to engage in sexual immorality impregnated that girl, will you follow the path of Cain and kill that unborn ‹d? Will you Run away, reject responsibility for your actions, or say concerning ‹ young lady like Cain, '*Am I my Brother's Keeper?*' She should have been more ‹ful; she seduced me. I am not the only one she has slept with. She should have ‹wed me to use a condom – all such voices would only compound our sins.

Some people have erroneously thought that those were the end of Cain's ‹ishments. Let's delve deeper.

When the descendants of Adam were listed, Cain's name was omitted. In ‹er words – he lost his inheritance. Across all the verses, one thing also comes ‹ strongly - All the descendants of Adam through Seth always had a Son and other ‹dren, ending with Noah, who was saved from the flood with his three sons.

*When Adam was 130 years old, he had a son who was like him, and he ‹ned him Seth;* **he had other children**. *When Seth was 105, he had a son, Enosh, ‹ then lived another 807 years. He* **had other children** *and died at the age of ‹. When Enosh was 90, he had a Son, Kenan. He* **had other children**. *When*

*Kenan was 70, he had a Son, Mahalalel **he had other children.** Noah had t*
***sons***.... ' *(Gen5:632)*

*Compare this genealogy with that of Cain:*

*"Cain and his wife had a son named Enoch. Then, Cain built a city named it after his son. Enoch had **a son** named Irad, who was the Fathe Mehujael, and Mehujael had **a son** named Methushael, who was the fathe. Lamech. **Lamech had two wives**, Adah and Zillah. Adah gave birth to Jabal, was the ancestor of those who raised livestock and lived in tents. His brother Jubal, the ancestor of all musicians who play the harp and the flute. Zillah g birth to Tubal Cain, who made all kinds of tools out of bronze and iron. Lam said to his wives, **I had killed** a young man because he struck me (Gen.4:17-24*

Could this be a mistake and, perchance, a modest way of listin genealogy? No, this text is correctly written. Compared with other genealog texts in the Bible, most times their children and other children are mentioned a Genesis 11:10-26 and Gen.10. Indeed, Cain struggled to bear children, which contrary to God's word in

Psalm 27: *Behold, children are a heritage from the Lord, the fruit of womb a **reward**. Blessed is the man whose quiver is full of them*;

Cain was so elated to finally bear a son that he named a whole city after son. His son and the generations after him struggled with childlessness and mos ended up with only one child. They began to build memorials and monume (cities, livestock, tents, and music) as achievements in place of the children t lacked. The blood of Abel so spoke against the lineage of Cain that the f polygamist and second recorded murder also came from his descendants.

How often do many families struggle with childlessness, miscarriag single children, and evil vices (smoking, drinking, murder, fornication, etc.) just because their lineage has ood on their hands'? How many times do you think you have sufficiently covered ır sins only to see the consequences of blood spilled begin to rear its ugly head our home and lineage? I pray that your lineage shall be delivered from blood lt in Jesus' Name, Amen.

Please do note that this is not to say all childless families have committed rtions or murdered someone. It is, however, important for such families to begin ing questions about their ancestors and genuinely give their lives to Jesus Christ l then pray against any blood that may be speaking against their lineage.

## David and Uriah – Amnon, Tamar, Absalom and Adonijah (2 m 11 - )

David – a man after God's own heart, decided to stay back home on a day ıgs were meant to go to war. He strolled on the balcony of his palace and saw an :eptionally beautiful woman having her bath in her house - Bathsheba. David ıt for her and had carnal knowledge of her (Sex) even though he was informed ıt the lady was married to one of his mighty soldiers who was deeply loyal to vid's reign. However, a few weeks later, she was pregnant, and in a bid to cover sin – he manipulated his way for her husband to sleep with her to no avail and entually ordered that Uriah.

(Bathsheba's husband) be murdered in Battle – David made Uriah deliver own death warrant by His own hand – **David's hands became stained with** ood. When David heard that Uriah was dead, he called for Bathsheba and made r his wife. This act sorely displeased God, and He sent Nathan, the Prophet, to liver judgment to David.

The consequences led to the death of the child and spilled over to lineage. Amnon, one of David's sons, suddenly developed a strange affection his half-sister – Tamar raped her and refused to marry her. Her brother – Absal heard of the ordeal and, for two whole years, plotted against and finally ki Amnon. Years later, Absalom became interested in the throne of his father, Da and attacked him, forcing David to flee his palace for several years. Absalom furt made things worse by openly fornicating with all of David's wives and concubi on the rooftop. Joab finally killed Absalom – David's Army commander.

After David's death, Uriah's blood kept speaking. Adonijah, one of Davi eldest sons, expressed interest in the Kingly throne by indirectly asking to ma one of David's concubines. Outraged - Solomon, his brother, killed Adonij Eventually, God refused David from building Him a temple because of his blo stained hands and instead transferred that privilege to his son – Solom Surprisingly, most of Bathsheba was mentioned in the Bible, even after husband's death – the Bible kept calling her 'the Wife of Uriah". Uriah's bl spoke through David's lineage.

## Saul and the Prophets' death

Saul was opportune to be the first King of Israel, but because he desi honor from his people more than pleasing God, he disobeyed God. The L rejected him and replaced him with young David. How often does peer press compel us to fall away from the grace of God? He became jealous of David a sought to kill him. At a time, he was informed that David was seen in the land the Priests called Nob – where he went to inquire of the Lord. Saul was enrag and spilled the blood of God's servants, not just the Priests but their famili including infants.

*Then the king ordered the guards at his side: "Turn and kill the priests of LORD because they too have sided with David. They knew he was fleeing, yet ʋ did not tell me." But the king's officials were unwilling to raise a hand to strike priests of the LORD.*

*[18] The king then ordered Doeg, "You turn and strike down the priests." So ɔg the Edomite turned and struck them down. That day, he killed eighty-five men ɔ wore the linen ephod. [19] He also put to the sword Nob, the town of the priests, h its men and women, its children and **infants**, and its cattle, donkeys, and sheep. Sam 22:17-19)*

Oh, how loudly the blood of these sacred people and children cried against l. One day, Saul was later killed in battle with three of his sons (1 Sam.31), luding Jonathan, but that was not all. In spite of Jonathan's kindness to David, too, was taken up in death. A few years later, Saul's entire generation was almost ɔed out, apart from Mephibosheth (Saul's grandson), who was lame on both feet, s spared. Even the deep mourning of the Prophet Samuel for Saul could not erse the consequences of his actions (1 Sam.16:1). In the word of Saul's ʋersaries, blood spoke more loudly to them than gold or silver.

*"Our quarrel with Saul and his family can't be settled with silver or gold, ⸱ do we want to kill any Israelite … "Saul wanted to destroy us and leave none of alive anywhere in Israel. [6] So hand over seven of his male descendants, and we 'l hang them before the LORD at Gibeah, the hometown of Saul, the LORD's chosen g" (2 Sam.21:4).*

The stains of blood are much too scarlet red to set apart the guilty from the ɔocent in vengeance. There is something about blood that ravages anything that nds on its path to vengeance.

# The heathen King and Son's sacrifice

Sometimes, we wonder why fetish persons are required to engage in blc rituals – this is because its potency is recognized in the spiritual realm. Their effe are as potent as their deadly consequences. Young people should, therefore, ce all manner of blood oath cult initiation requiring blood and blood sacrifices. Ne be lured ever to consider this because the *life of a creature is in the blood, an have given it to you to make atonement for yourselves on the altar; it is the blc that makes atonement for one's life (Lev.17:11).*

*"When the king of Moab saw that the battle had gone against him, he tc with him seven hundred swordsmen to break through to the king of Edom, but th failed. [27] Then he took his firstborn son, who was to succeed him as king and offe. him as a sacrifice on the city wall. The fury against Israel was great; they withdr and returned to their own land"* (2 Kings 3:26-27).

God had earlier warned the Israelites never to pass their children throu fire/sacrifice (Lev.18:21)– a form of cult worship of idols. This Moabite Ki Mesha, considering that he would obviously lose the battle to Judah and Edom, w had allied against him, quickly took his son (his successor to the throne) a sacrificed him on the city wall to the god Chemosh in full view of his adversari This evil act aroused divine anger amongst his opponents, but it sure turned the back, thereby restraining them from conquering his Kingdom. This is the poten of blood.

**Saul of Tarsus** In the book of the Acts of the Apostles, Saul witness Stephen's death while he gave his support. Eventually, the Lord Jesus Christ call Saul to be a witness to Christianity after his name was changed to Paul. It is wo noting that amidst Saul's zeal for the Lord, he suffered more than all the apost (2 Corinthians 11:16 – 33), and the Jews rejected him. His greatest missiona

gress was amongst the Gentile nations considered by the Jews as 'those who are
out.'

## 7. Levitical standards of blood

In Levitical times, mainly governed by the mosaic law, there were three
s sin was atoned for, and all required blood. First, a goat is gotten (the
egoat), and the whole congregation will confess their sins on the goat and send
vay into the forest, where it would most likely be devoured.

Second, everyone was to bring an animal to the temple, burn the fat, and
r it to the Lord, preferably the best of the sheep or a dove for low-income
ilies (Lev.15:15, Lev 16, Lev.17). Third, which is a typology of Christ's
itual intervention, the Priest is to enter into the Holy of Holies once a year where
ark of the Lord is kept, and he is to atone first for his sins and that of the people
prinkling the blood of the sacrificed animal on the altar after he has taken part
he ceremonial cleansing. A rope and a bell are tied to his waist so that when
ring the sacrifice of an animal if the Lord (who does not behold iniquity) strikes
 to death if he is not qualified, the inactive bell will notify the people that he is
d. He will be dragged out with the rope.

For the life of a creature is in the blood, and I have given it to you to make
nement for yourselves on the altar; it is the blood that makes atonement for one's
. **12** So I tell the people of Israel this: "None of you may eat blood, and no
eigner living among you may eat blood." **13** "If any citizen of Israel or foreigner
ng among you catches a wild animal or bird that can be eaten, that person must
r the blood on the ground and cover it with dirt."**14** If blood is still in the meat,
animal's life is still in it. So I give this command to the people of Israel: "Don't

eat meat that still has blood in it, because the animal's life is in its blood. Any
who eats blood must be cut off."(Lev.17:11-14)

## Is Blood Transfusion a Sin?

In a bid to compress all the Levitical laws guiding blood, after Jesus's de
the only requirement regarding this subject was.

"It is my judgment, therefore, that we should not make it difficult for
Gentiles who are turning to God. Instead, we should write to them, telling then
abstain from food polluted by idols, from sexual immorality, from the mea
strangled animals, and from blood. **(Acts 15: 19-21)**

By Jewish standards, an animal will be beheaded entirely or slit throu
and the animal hung upside down to completely allow the blood to drain from
animal before they are now thoroughly cooked for eating. This is a good prac
that most Christians have also imbibed by slitting the throats of animals, but m
Christians do not entirely allow the blood to drain. Some sects, such as
Jehovah's Witnesses, have rejected all forms of blood, including denouncing bl
transfusion. But is this really God's intention? God must intend to save a lif
which is the ultimate intent of Christ's death on the cross.

No matter how much blood is drained from an animal, there are still tra
of blood found in the meat and bone marrow, but we go ahead and eat the meat a
cooking. When a farmer who rears chicken or other animals sees one of their l
bruised or broken and emitting blood, the farmer of today, who may be a Jehova
Witness, will immediately bind that leg so the animal will not die. These are ma
other ways we come in contact with blood that do not make it sinful. How mu
more Blood transfusion, especially when it is geared to save a life – it is not sin
In two instances, Jesus Christ provided strong examples of why we must see

her truth when applying the laws, such as when it would help save a life. In the
saic law, It was abominable for a lady emitting blood of any kind, especially
ing her menstrual flow, to come in contact with other people or, worse still, a
phet. Hence, women were banished from coming to the temple when they were
emonially unclean. But the woman with the issue of blood had suffered many
ngs in the hands of doctors, had given up on a medical cure, and may die, but she
ched the hem of Jesus's garment, and she was healed. Jesus did not condemn
. Instead, he blessed her. Another example is the Pharisees murmured when Jesus
led a woman who was bent over for 18 years because he healed her on the
bath. Jesus said something, **15** The Lord answered him, *"You hypocrites!*
*esn't each of you on the Sabbath untie your ox or donkey from the stall and lead*
*ut to give it water? 16 Then should not this woman, a daughter of Abraham,*
*om Satan has kept bound for eighteen long years, be set free on the Sabbath day*
*m what bound her?" Luke 13:10-17.* Something similar also happened to a man
o was lame for 38 years and was healed by Jesus. It means that God values
man life more than ceremonial or religious laws. If we cannot make one life, then
should be willing to give a blood transfusion to save a life. Remember that the
son God commanded us to stay away from blood was because he wants us to be
althy, not to serve other gods, and to remain alive. If that law will make us kill a
e, then it is no longer from God.

*For you will be expelled from the synagogues, and the time is coming when*
*se who kill you will think they are doing a holy service for God. (John 16:2)*

Another important bible truth in this regard is the parable of the good
maritan (Luke 10:25 – 37). We should be curious as to why well-meaning and
spected people in the service of God, such as the Priest and Levite, would walk
st a man who has been beaten, wounded, obviously bleeding profusely and left
r dead without stopping to help. We should wonder why a Samaritan, who the

Jews regarded as less Jewish, would stop and clean the wounds of this half-d[...] man and then take him to an inn to receive care. The answers are in the Law[...] Moses. In the book of Leviticus, God, through Moses, outlined how the Israel[...] should live, especially the Priests and Levites. In fact, God had slain the sons[...] Aaron in the temple for offering strange fire during their ceremonial sacri[...] (Leviticus 10), and it became an example for all to revere the ordinances of G[...] Also, in Leviticus 15, God warned the Israelites to abstain from bodily flui[...] including semen and the menstrual blood of a woman. We can bet that the Pri[...] and Levite in Luke 10 were probably stuck on these ordinances because they [...] not want to be unclean to the point that they walked past a dying man with wou[...] and blood all over him. They were not even sure if he was still alive, yet they wo[...] still walk past because the Mosaic law had also said one would be unclean if[...] touched a dead person. The Priest and Levite actually thought they were doing G[...] a service by not saving a life, but Jesus Christ faulted their devotion and clea[...] praised the Samaritan for doing the right thing of saving a life instead of getti[...] stuck in laws that did not save lives.

If I am to echo Jesus's words today, I would say – "You religious hypocrit[...] if you can eat that meat/chicken that has some strains of blood in it or bone marro[...] if you can bind an animal's wounded legs just to preserve the life of that chick[...] or animal how much more save the life of a human being who requires blood [...] live."

Jesus Christ also died and shed his blood for our sins so that we may g[...] eternal life. Unfortunately, many have ignorantly let blood on their hands in t[...] guise of not transfusing blood. The verdict

*If I warn the wicked, saying, 'You are under the penalty of death,' but y[...] fail to deliver the warning, they will die in their sins. And I will hold you responsi[...] for their deaths. (Eze.3:18)*

Yes, it is important to note that people can transfer sicknesses and diseases ough blood transfusion. A father who was in his window period of HIV infection ated blood to his sick daughter, but the tests could not detect the virus due to its dow period. Still, the daughter was later diagnosed as HIV positive. It is, refore, crucial that blood donations be thoroughly subjected to all medical eening before transfusing. Nevertheless, this should not be a reason to prohibit od completely.

**How to Prevent Teen and Unplanned Pregnancy**

⊙ Abstinence: Virginity (A rare treasure): Abstinence is the most effective way to prevent an unplanned pregnancy, especially for teenagers. As morals erode in our society, it is still worth noting that the value of virginity is still a rare and valuable treasure that, when lost, can never be recovered.

⊙ Do not let a crush fester – Proverbs 4:23. As young people mature physically/biologically, and emotionally, you will often get drawn to the opposite gender at some point, which is natural. Some may be borne from a genuine admiration of someone's skills, looks, demeanor, or character. Nevertheless, spending long hours daydreaming about your crush may lead you to seek ways to be with them, spend more time with and eventually lead you to rationalize indulgences such as pecking, necking, kissing, and smooching, which may dangerously lead one to sexual intimacy. Instead, practice the art of self-discipline right from your heart. When the thoughts come, decide to divert them to other productive activities like reading, engaging in sports, or events that will keep your heart from lust.

The story in 2 Samuel 13 about Amnon and his half-sister Tamar is a ngent reminder of the long-term consequences of an uncontrolled desire/crush.

- Set healthy boundaries with the opposite gender (avoid spending too m...
  time or smooching)

- Engage your mind and activities in healthy activities

- Avoid pornography

- Ask an adult or social worker for answers to your nagging questi...
  anytime you are in doubt.

- The use of contraceptives can be an option for those who are alre...
  sexually active and unable to abstain; however, there are various types
  contraceptives, and you must talk to a sexual health professional or Doc
  for the most suitable one for your body.

Also, bear in mind that biblically, the intention of using contraceptives
important to God. The story of Onan and Tamar in the Bible (Genesis 38) sho
the tragic end of a man who used the withdrawal method of contraception becau
he had a sinister motive.

**Ethical Issues in Fertility Procedures such as Assisted Reproducti**
**Therapy as In-vitro Fertilization (IVF) and Surrogacy**

**Surrogacy** is an arrangement, often supported by a legal agreeme
whereby a woman (the surrogate mother) agrees to bear a child for another pers
or persons who will become the child's parent(s) after birth. Globally, there is
steady increase in demand for surrogacy, especially to tackle infertility (Peras:
2018). Christian bioethicists agree that most forms of ART, especially surroga
are laden with issues because, theologically and morally, they bother on t
exploitation of women (for example, womb renting in surrogacy), interference
the marriage covenant by introducing a third party (surrogate or egg donor), sale

nts (high costs of surrogacy) and most importantly the use of embryo-ructive reproductive technology (discarding of unused embryos).

Although the Bible does not mention or forbid surrogacy, the closest the e mentioned were in the cases of Hagar bearing a child for Sarah and when ecca had asked Jacob to go into her maid Bilhah to have children for her. In e two cases, it was laden with heartaches. For Hagar, it seemed increasingly cult for her to completely detach from Ishmael, ultimately leading to pain, tache, and confusion. This can still happen today, as women discover that ng away their children (despite financial compensation) can cause easurable pain because of the bond that forms between the pregnant mother the child she is carrying, even before it is born. In addition, many surrogates arely fully informed of the long and arduous journey to surrogacy characterized nental, physical, and emotional stress and the number of hormonal injections will have to receive during the process. Many also do not know that God gned the female body to bond with the child in the womb emotionally, nonally, and biologically. Sometimes, a couple may feel obligated to go the a mile for a surrogate and raise questions of conscience. The Bible states that dren are gifts and not rights (Psalm 127:3). Just as God blesses some persons 1 wealth, intellect, and unique gifts, so does he also bless others with children. ples who are unable to have children should not act in outright defiance of 's leading because they see it as a right to have children. Instead, they should erfully consider the option only if they have the peace from God to forge on 1 surrogacy or even IVF as a viable alternative. Remember that *"Whatever you or drink or whatever you do, you must do all for the glory of God"*

*orinthians 10:31).*

The fall of man created lots of problems, including infertility, and this es God sad. God has provided science to solve human problems, and so far, it does not violate divine principles of the preservation of human life (embryos) the marital bond. Surrogacy may look like an option for childlessness, but a clo look reveals that it may open even more doors to confusion and heartache. Child couples can go through a lot of emotional pain but should realize that all thi work together for good (even childlessness) for those who fear God (Rom.8: Jesus Christ is calling us daily to *"Come to me, all you who are weary and burder and I will give you rest. Take my yoke upon you and learn from me, for I am ge and humble in heart, and you will find rest for your souls. (Matt.11:28-29)* (P. 1998)

## Surrogacy around the world

- Thailand, Nepal, Mexico, and India have all recently banned foreign commercial surrogacy.

- Several countries, including France, Germany, Italy, and Spain, prohibit surrogacy in all forms.

- In countries including the UK, Ireland, Denmark, and Belgium, surrogacy is allowed only when the surrogate is not paid or only paid for reasonable expenses.

## The Grey Area/Ethical Issue in the IVF Process

In this light, there is a procedure during in-vitro fertilization (IVF - a method ed to address infertility) that requires the fertilization of follicles extracted from ovaries using sperm cells. Sometimes, as many as Ten to twelve embryos are tilized through this process, but only very few, as little as two or three, are erted back into the woman's uterus, believing there would be implantation. metimes, the remaining embryos are discarded or used for research purposes – s also is abortion and the deliberate termination of life. It is recommended that dical personnel harvest fewer eggs with the most viability, and patients should nsider freezing their embryos for use later in life rather than discarding them. ost importantly, embryo donation/adoption should be encouraged as an ernative.

On average, only about 25 percent of embryos that are created using IVF d transferred to the womb develop until birth. Because of this high failure rate, F often involves creating more embryos than will be implanted in the womb. The ibryos are usually kept in a state of suspended animation (i.e., cryogenically frozen) until their death (which usually occurs in less than 10 years). Seve passages in the Bible strongly suggest that human life begins at conception (. 31:13-15; Psalms 51:5; 139:13-16; Matthew 1:20). The Bible is also clear about taking of innocent life (Exodus 20:13; Deuteronomy. 5:17). For these reaso Christians should not support any reproductive techniques that create embryos t will not be implanted in a womb. One surrogacy arrangement that some Christ bioethicists believe may at times be morally acceptable is "rescue surrogacy," wl a surrogate mother volunteers her womb to save an IVF-created embryo that l been frozen and is destined for destruction (Carter, 2017), otherwise known embryo adoption.

**Rescue surrogacy/Embryo Adoption** can be the answer to this proble These embryos can be donated to other couples to adopt them and be transplan into other women who may be battling infertility. For sanctity's sake, we recommend this route instead of those embryos to be discarded, which tantamount to abortion. Many Medical practitioners may disagree with this, but Government is encouraged to set policies that can encourage life and regulate practices of Fertility clinics to adopt saner methods of embryo manageme Remember, in natural fertilization, the human body releases only one ovum : fertilization per month and, in rare conditions, two. Even God designed the hum body to preserve lives.

God is deeply in love with children and spells doom for anyone w misleads them - But Jesus said,

"Let the children come to me. Don't stop them! For the Kingdom of Heav belongs to those who are like these children." (Mtt.19:14). "But whoever causes t downfall of one of these little ones who believe in Me--it would be better for h if a heavy millstone were hung around his neck and he were drowned in the dep of the sea! (Mtt.18:6 – HCSB)

## The final and Most Effective Remedy for Blood spill

Why Must God Spill Blood to forgive Sin and not merely Forgive?

Because blood speaks and cries vengeance anytime it is taken forcefully. *n the LORD said: Why have you done this terrible thing? You killed your own ther, and his blood flowed onto the ground. Now, his blood is calling out for me unish you. (Gen.4:10).*

*Rom.6:23:* For the wages of sin is death, but the gift of God is eternal life Christ Jesus our Lord.

## Abraham a typology of Jesus' death

The familiar Abraham's story is one of great faith and patience in the Lord he sought a child. After God finally blessed him at the age of 99, one day, when child was growing up, God asked Abraham to sacrifice his son.

"Take your son, your only son—yes, Isaac, whom you love so much—and to the land of Moriah. Go and sacrifice him as a burnt offering on one of the untains, which I will show you." (Gen.22:2)

"**Abraham** believed **God, and it was credited** to him as **righteousness**." en.15:6). God wanted to test Abraham's heart. He would never allow Abraham kill Isaac physically because, by nature, God hated murder. Many years after raham's act, God warned the Israelites never to pass their children through the e/sacrifice (Lev.18:21). Although Abraham had not yet been given this unction, he nevertheless was willing to offer his Son until God stopped him and ked him instead to offer an animal. Isaac lived on to an old age. God had planned sacrifice his only Son, Jesus Christ, to save the world. It was a difficult plan for

God, yet only Jesus was qualified (Rev.5:1-7), and He gave us Jesus for our sak
Throughout the scriptures, only Abraham was willing to pay the kind of sacrif
God madeto save mankind. No wonder he is called the 'Father of Many Nation

As a young person, what would you sacrifice to keep your chastity or t
unplanned pregnancy for the sake of God? Would you trust God to provide for t
child? Would you be willing to go through the rigors of motherhood, the sacrif
of shame, the risk of skipping a year or two in school, the loneliness just to sa
that child just to avoid blood on your hands and because God said so? The rewa
- *He who did not spare his own son, but gave him up for us all--how will he*
*also, along with him, graciously give us all things? (Rom.8:32)* including life.

## Jesus Christ, the High Priest of our Salvation

An excerpt from the sayings of Late Pst. Ravi Zacharias (June 25, 201
captures the need to grasp what Jesus did for us. Like 5,000 years ago, Abraha
took up his son to be sacrificed, but God kept Abraham's hands from bringing do
that Axe to harm his boy because God promised him that He would provide
sacrifice for himself. Three thousand years later, God fulfilled that promise; he to
His only Son, Jesus Christ, to the hill of Golgotha to be sacrificed for the salvati
of the world, and this time the Axe did not stop. Jesus Christ died on the Cross
Calvary; it was a painful, voluntary, and glorious death that finally broke the pow
of sin, addiction, and death in the life of anyone who accepted that gift. Until
accept and receive the Son that God has sent in Jesus Christ, we will keep offeri
our unborn Sons and daughters on the abortion table for honor, position, power, a
prestige. Except you genuinely receive the offer of God in our hearts, you will ke
offering your bodies on the altar of fornication and adultery yet ultimately wish
run from the consequences of that sinful action.

When Christ came as high Priest of the good things that are already here, he
t through the greater and more perfect Tabernacle that is not man-made, that is
ay, not a part of this creation. He did not enter by means of the blood of goats
calves, but he entered the Most Holy Place once and for all by his own blood,
ing obtained eternal redemption. The blood of goats and bulls and the ashes of
ifer sprinkled on those who are ceremonially unclean sanctify them so that they
outwardly clean. How much more, then, will the blood of Christ, who through
eternal Spirit offered himself unblemished to God, cleanse our consciences from
that lead to death so that we may serve the living God! **Hebrews 9:11-14**

## 8. What if it looks like the consequences of one's actions are still nifest even after they are born again?

Dave was young and vibrant; however, due to his upbringing, he found
self in a gang, leading him to kill a young, innocent girl who was deaf and
nb. With time, he gave his life to Christ and got married; God would later bless
m with a baby girl. However, all attempts for his wife to conceive again proved
rtive. He would look through his past and wonder if he was suffering the
sequences of his actions.

Many have done so many atrocities willfully, not fearing God, and when the
sequences of their actions show up, they run to church to be saved; yes, they
l be saved. However, many get so bloated with pride and a sense of entitlement,
e the proud Pharisee in (Luke 18:9-14) by consistently quoting I am now a new
ature, old things have passed away behold all things have become new Lord give
that blessing, heal me, bless me with children and give me my dreams. They
use to patiently wait for God to show his mercy by removing the consequences
h time; they forget the scriptures quickly:

*Do not be deceived, for whatsoever a man sows, he will reap, for ( cannot be mocked.*

The same goes for millions of Christians and couples out there go through childlessness and strange issues in their marriage even after they are b again. Unfortunately, no one knows why God shows mercy and Grace to cer people and why some do not receive it. Two girls go to the same party – they li rough life, both commit abortions they get married – one struggles to have child the other receives mercy and gets her heart desires, including children. It even g trickier – a young girl lives a sexually loose life; she never gets pregnant all thro her escapades, whereas the virgin God-fearing girl decides to sleep with boyfriend one day, and boom – she is pregnant, only one sexual act. Does this m God is unrighteous? No.

Another scripture gives a clue that those who fear the Lord are more lik to obtain mercy from him:

*"AND HIS MERCY IS UPON GENERATION AFTER GENERATION TOWARD THOSE W FEAR HIM. (Luke 1:50)*

David was a man after God's own heart, but God said

I will be his Father, and he will be My son. When he does wrong, I v discipline *him with the rod of men and with the blows of the sons of men. But* loving devotion will never depart from him as I removed it from Saul, whor moved out of your way. *Your house and kingdom will endure forever before N and your throne will be established forever."…(2 Sam 7:14-16)*

Paul was an apostle of Christ and had sorely persecuted the Christia before his conversion. He personally monitored the death of Stephen and stood a witness for Christians to be killed (Acts 22:20), then went from town to tov dragging out Christians and putting them in Prison. He was such a terror to

ristian community that even after his conversion, Ananias was afraid to go and
.y for him. However, Paul encountered Jesus Christ on one of such trips and then
Idenly faced so much persecution compared to other disciples and apostles of
us.

*23 Are they servants of Christ? (I am out of my mind to talk like this.) I am
re. I have worked much harder, been in prison more frequently, been flogged
re severely, and been exposed to death again and again. 24 Five times I received
m the Jews the forty lashes minus one. 25 Three times I was beaten with rods,
ce I was pelted with stones, three times I was shipwrecked, I spent a night and a
v in the open sea, 26 I have been constantly on the move. I have been in danger
m rivers, in danger from bandits, in danger from my fellow Jews, in danger from
ntiles; in danger in the city, in danger in the country, in danger at sea, and in
nger from false believers. 27 I have labored and toiled and have often gone
hout sleep; I have known hunger and thirst and have often gone without food; I
ve been cold and naked. 28 Besides everything else, I face daily the pressure of
concern for all the churches. 29 Who is weak, and I do not feel weak? Who is led
o sin, and I do not inwardly burn? (2 Corinthians 11:23-29 (NIV)*

The truth is, there is a difference between forgiveness of sins and Mercy
it removes the consequences of our actions, otherwise known as Grace. When a
l fornicates and gets pregnant, if she gives her life to Jesus Christ, it doesn't make
e pregnancy go away; she will still need to deliver the baby and care for the child
th so much love. The same goes for someone who contracts an incurable Sexually
ansmitted Disease (STD). When he truly gets born again and gives his life to
sus Christ, he is forgiven, but it does not make the STD go away. It is only in
bmission to God's will to suffer with Christ through our hardships willingly does
od shows mercy. What is mercy? Mercy is the prerogative of God to forgive
meone and mercifully take away the consequences of their actions even though

they do not deserve it. Jesus Christ forgave the woman who was bent over for 18 whom Satan had bound; He forgave and healed the man who was sick/lame on bed for 38years; he also forgave the adulterous woman with a charge – 'Go and no more,' then the Lord can surely show mercy and take away the consequences our action. But what is certain in the scripture is this –

*"Come now, let's settle this," says the LORD. "Though your sins are scarlet, I will make them as white as snow. Though they are red like crimson, I make them as white as wool (Isi.1:18).*

God's forgiveness is sure – we will not die spiritually; when the trump sounds, we will ultimately be with him in heaven – which is the greatest goal of Christian; however, here on earth is not our home, and the consequences of actions may turn around to haunt us in the cloak of persecutions and trials – *Con it all joy when you pass through diverse temptation, for the testing of our faith h been tried by fire...* Grace or Mercy is unmerited favor – it means when we dese to be punished, yet he mercifully or graciously gives us a blessing we do deserve. It is when we have done evil and deserve to be punished spiritually physically, but Jesus Christ shows up and takes it on himself for our sake. Howev Mercy is not a sure deal in the path of salvation. As harsh as it sounds, it is tru the Bible says

"14 What then shall we say? Is God unjust? Certainly not! For He says Moses: "I will have mercy on whom I have mercy, and I will have compassion whom I have compassion." So then, it does not depend on man's desire or eff but on God's mercy."(Romans 9:15-16).

And He said, "I Myself will make all My goodness pass before you and proclaim the name of the LORD before you, and I will be gracious to whom I be gracious and will show compassion on whom I will show compassio (Exo.33:19)

So then He has mercy on whom He desires, and He hardens whom He ires. (Rom.9:18)

Anytime the Lord goes further to speak not only of forgiveness of sins but toring physical blessings - mercy and compassion are at work.

When the LORD will have compassion on Jacob and again choose Israel, and le them in their own land, then strangers will join them and attach themselves he house of Jacob. **Ezekiel39:25**

Therefore thus says the Lord GOD, "Now I will restore the fortunes of Jacob l have mercy on the whole house of Israel; and I will be jealous for My holy ne. **Psalm102:13**

You will arise and have compassion on Zion; For it is time to be gracious to , For the appointed time has come.

When we repent, our sins are forgiven, but there is a time when the Lord nself will arise for us to smite our enemies, restore all that the cankerworm has en, and physically turn away the reproach and consequences of our actions. It mes not by us just demanding it but by being patient in tribulation, trials and rsecutions while praying for his mercies to prevail.


## GOD'S LOVE TO THE SINNER

**Isaiah 1:18:** "Come now, let us settle the matter," says the LORD. "Though ur sins are like scarlet, they shall be as white as snow; though they are red as mson, they shall be like wool.

**Psalm 32:1:** "Blessed is the one whose transgressions are forgiven, whose is are covered." 1 John 1:9: "If we confess our sins, he is faithful and just to rgive us our sins and to cleanse us from all unrighteousness.

**Hebrews 8:12 says,** "For I will forgive their wickedness and will remem▮ their sins no more.

**Psalm 103 says 12:** "As far as the east is from the west, so far has removed our transgressions from us.

**Daniel 9:9** "The Lord our God is merciful and forgiving, even though ` have rebelled against him."

**Isaiah 43:25:** "I, even I, am he who blots out your transgressions, for ▮ own sake, and remembers your sins no more ..."

**Ephesians 1:7-8** "In Him we have redemption through His blood, ▮ forgiveness of sins, according to the riches of His grace which He made to abou▮ toward us in all wisdom and prudence."

# Options for Unplanned Pregnancies

Married and unmarried women who find they are pregnant may begin to onsider if they have an idea to abort. Today, there are several options that can be lored without spilling blood or resorting to abortion. Options include:

You may decide to give birth and parent your baby: This comes with a huge ponsibility – a stable income, time to dedicate to the child's learning, growth, e, and companionship. There are many single moms who have taken on this ture, and they have found it rewarding. There are many charities and community ncies that provide support for single mothers.

Adoption: Carrying the baby to term and giving the child up to couples who unable to have biological children of their own. The first option for many ples seeking children of their own but unable to is usually adoption. However, ny couples across several countries have reported more difficulty and lengthier es to get matched with a birth mother/baby. Many have been forced into child ficking, which is a crime under local and international laws. It is important to ister with the appropriate agency of your Country in charge of adoption issues. re are also non-profit agencies that are involved with legal international ption. There are agencies that have the legal authority and ethical boundaries to age in the adoption process. These agencies are usually there from pregnancy doption and even post-partum support. Note that for adoption, the child will se to become yours legally, and all parental rights will be given to the adoptive ents.

Fostering: If you do not wish to give up your child for outright adoption, tering may be an option. This is when someone would help to bring up your baby a period that you all will mutually agree upon to return and reclaim the child; it ld be short-term or long-term fostering. For students who desire to complete their education or an unemployed person seeking a stable job before taking on huge responsibility of caring for a child, fostering may be a better option. Fo: parents may or may not be close relatives, however, it is important to either invc an agency with the responsibility of monitoring the process or have clear te: before starting your fostering journey. Remember that foster parents will eventu: develop a strong bond with your child, and the kind of morals you want the cl to imbibe all influence this process. Anyone can foster a child. However, pec may prioritize a family unit with a Father and Mother figure and those who alre: have children of their own, which can make the child reclaiming process : emotionally difficult. Not everyone may have the perfect conditions for fosterir

## Proposed Bill Resolutions

In the light of the difficulties confronting adoption, lawmakers encouraged to push for these legislations:

Adoption should not be the only active and viable option open to the b: mother, but a mother haven carried a baby for 9 months and formed a bond w that child should be given the option of accepting the baby back and given suffici time to reclaim that child.

If she is unable to cater to the child at the moment, institutional care sho be provided for her and her baby for a minimum of 3 to 6 months.

A maximum of 10 years and a minimum of 3 years should be given to mother to return back to reclaim her child, knowing that long-term institutio support is not in the best interest of any child.

A foster parent should be made to follow up and possibly care for the ch if the exit time for the child from the institutional home has elapsed.

Foster parents must have children of their own of both sexes and be willing relinquish the child to the biological mother when she returns.

However, in cases where the biological mother has vehemently refused to ep the child nor come back for the child even after birth, especially if she has er children before now, the child can be given up for adoption to caring, stable nilies, preferably with a mother and father figure.

## Proposed intervention for infertile couples

We are enjoined to empathize with couples who are yet to have their own ldren.

However, both gestational and traditional surrogacy, for reasons spelled out ove in the text, may not be the recommended option.

It is recommended that regulations guiding Assisted Reproductive chnology (ART), such as IVF and Artificial insemination, be reviewed. ART ould be legally approved only when all fertilized embryos will be transferred to emale body for implantation possibly through embryo donation.

- IVF procedures accompanied by discarding fertilized embryos should be abolished as life begins at conception.
- Couples should have the option of donating their unneeded embryos to interested couples (especially infertile couples) to carry them to term in a loving and stable family unit through a term called 'embryo adoption.' Thanks to many clinics who are already offering these services.
- Everyone who is willing, medically fit, in a socially acceptable age or marital status to carry a baby to term should be allowed to adopt embryos.

- Rescue surrogacy/embryo adoption is the willingness and ability to ca[rry] fertilized fresh/frozen embryos to term by either biological/non-biologi[cal] parents and delivered in cases where they would have been discarded [or] used for scientific purposes.

- The world must begin to look towards rescue surrogacy as a panacea to [the] rising rate of infertility in the world rather than the high expectations of [live] birth adoption.

- Adoption of rescue surrogacy for infertile couples would be m[ore] meaningful, create a deeper sense of bond between child and couples, a[nd] still carry a deeper feeling of motherhood for infertile couples than [the] traditional adoption method.

# What is the Price?
# True Story of a Teen now a Mother

You may be wondering what this question means. Price of what? I will tell you. Kindly read my story before you decide about your pregnancy.

When I was 17 years old, I got pregnant. I thought about the price I would pay – having a child out of wedlock, missing significant time from school to have the baby, possibly dropping out from University, the ridicule from the public, the disappointment from my parents, especially my Dad – he so believed in me to make the family proud and I was the most academically inclined among all of his children because I got admission to the University at the age of 15 years and started at 16, loved that I was always indoors to attend to him when I was home, I was reserved; the price of losing my esteem, the price of having a baby for a man I did not love and may never get married to, the price tags were pretty costly, enough to rule out the possibility of keeping the baby. Strangely, it seemed like a smooth sail. No one surprisingly challenged me to brace up to the price nor to strongly consider other options. The clinic only asked me to bring in my mum to give her consent, which she willingly did (yes, even my mum – that authority figure only expressed her disappointment but never told me to reconsider the decision to abort the baby). Within minutes, it was done surgically, and I returned to school after a few days; it did not stop me from having unprotected sex with my new boyfriend; I only got scared of getting pregnant, which made me take emergency contraceptives at will. I would later graduate with almost a distinction at the age of 20 years– worth it, right?

By 26, I was happily married but unable to have children. Within 13 years marriage, I had undergone 5 IVF procedures and 2 blighted ovum miscarriages.

We were unable to adapt, and for years, I regretfully thought about my nai
teenage decision. Looking back, I wish I had been encouraged to consider otl
options. If someone had fostered that child for me, I would have happily welcom
him/her back into my life, not only because we struggled to have children t
because, now that I am older, I know better. I know anyone (either in the family
outside) would have been willing to groom the child. I now know that I would'
been able to remain in school to have the child or go to a private place for a fe
months to have the baby without anyone knowing; I know I would've still be
able to make good grades, I know any man who loves me will be willing to stick
me and still marry me irrespective of my past, I now know that my Dad might ha
been disappointed, but he would still love me, most importantly I know that I wou
have given that child a chance to live, grow and look into my eyes someday to s
– "Thank you that you did not let me die" – it would have been the bravest decisi
that I ever took especially for the gift of life for an unborn child. Today, I have r
own children, but many do not understand the story behind my kids. It was
journey of heartache, tireless waiting, and cries. I went through the journey
seeing countless of my embryos retrieved and discarded; during one frozen embr
transfer, only two out of all my embryos were inserted, which did not lead
conception. Thankfully, we had a child out of all the IVF procedures until I realiz
the Lord was nudging me to wait on him. I decided to stop the IVFs and trust Gc
I just could not stand the thought of all those discarded embryos. The Lord hea
me; miraculously, I conceived naturally two times, and the children are doing we

I want to ask you – What cost do you consider too much to keep your bab
Why not reconsider the decision?

*Psalm 139: 13-16: For you created my inmost being, you knit me togeth*
*in my mother's womb. I praise you because I am fearfully and wonderfully maa*
*your works are wonderful; I know that full well. My frame was not hidden from yo*
*when I was made in the secret place when I was woven together in the depths of t*

*h. Your eyes saw my unformed body; all the days ordained for me were written*
*our book before one of them came to be.*

Is there a more sensitive issue you think is too hard to pay the price? Thank
for your decision to consider other options.

-Anonymous

# References

1. Abortion http://www.siue.edu/~evailat/el10.html

2. HOW to REPORT on ABORTION A guide for journalists, editors, and media outlets https://www.ippf.org/sites/default/files/2018-04/Media%20Guidelines%20on%20how%20to%20report%20on%20Abortion.pdf

3. Inequities in the incidence and safety of abortion in LMIC Suzanne O Bell, Elizabeth Omoluabi, Funmilola OlaOlorun, Mridula Shankar, Caroline Moreau http://orcid.org/0000-0002-8637-62491

4. Surrogate mothers: 'I gave birth, but it's not my baby' By Valeria Perasso (December 2018) https://www.bbc.com/news/world-46430250

5. Jim Paul (1998) Surrogacy - Christian Medical Fellowship https://www.google.com/search?sxsrf=ALeKk006_hJMZFQ8jBTddTD2P5NhPCXg%3A1603482084611&ei=5DGTX63iJOHFgwfolobwAw&q=surrogacy+and+christianity&oq=surrogacy+a+christianity&gs_lcp=CgZwc3ktYWIQAzIFCAAQyQM6BAgAEEc6BgjECc6BwgAEMkDEEM6BAgAEEM6AggAOgYIABAWEB5QjasKWzPCmDF0gpoAHADeACAAdMEiaHOL5IBCTItNS44LjIuMpgBAKABAaoBB2d3cy13aXrIAQjAAQE&sent=psyab&ved=0ahUKEwit5LmgvMvsAhXh4uAKHWiLAT4Q4dUDCA0&uact=5

6. Joe Carter (November 16, 2017 ) Basic Bioethics: What Christians should know about surrogacy. The Ethics and Religious Liberty Commission of the Southern Baptist Convention https://erlc.com/resource-library/articles/basicbioethics-what-christians-should-know-about-surrogacy/

7. Guttmacher Institute (2022) "Unintended Pregnancy and Abortion Worldwide" Global and Regional Estimates of Unintended Pregnancy and Abortion. Retrieved from https://www.guttmacher.org/fact-sheet/induced-abortionworldwide

www.ingramcontent.com/pod-product-compliance
Lightning Source LLC
Chambersburg PA
CBHW052123030426
42335CB00025B/3085